How to be more slender, less fatty and more grounded:

The Straightforward Study of building a definitive female body

By

Mary M. Bennett

Table of content

Basic ways of defining well-being and wellness objectives that will rouse you

Introduction

"Regardless of how bad you might think your hereditary qualities are, and regardless of how lost you could feel after attempting and forsaking many sorts of diets and exercises, you totally, positively can have the lean, provocative body that you long for".

Consider the possibility that I COULD Tell YOU the best way to decisively change your body quicker than you at any point expected. Imagine a scenario where I provided you with the specific recipe of activity and eating that makes losing 10 to 15 pounds of fat while likewise constructing fit muscle a breeze...and it would just require 10 to 12 weeks. Imagine a scenario where I told you the best way to get a conditioned, athletic build that you love is by effective money management, something like 5% of your time every day. Imagine a scenario in which I let you know that you can accomplish that "Hollywood darling" body without having your life rotate around it-no for extended periods in the rec centre, no destitute yourself, and no tiresome cardio that makes you feel sick. I'll try and tell you the best way to get inclined while yet enjoying the "cheat" food sources that you love consistently like pasta, pizza, and frozen yoghourt, imagine a scenario in which I vowed to be next to you the whole way, assisting you with staying away from the tricks, entanglements, and issues that a great many people fall into, assisting you with efficiently accomplishing your actual hereditary potential, and fundamentally giving my best for see you accomplish the best body you've at any point had. Suppose you got up each day, thoroughly searched in the mirror, and couldn't help but grin at your appearance. Envision the lift in certainty you'd feel if you did have that obstinate midsection and thigh far any longer and were no more "that one young lady" yet rather had lean, hot bends and were "that one young lady" Envision, only 12 weeks from now, being continually commended on what you look like and asked what on earth you're doing to gain such surprising headway with your body. Envision partaking in the additional advantages of having higher energy levels, better spirits, and less throbbing painfulness and of realising that you're getting better consistently. Indeed, you can have these things, and it's not close to as confounded as the wellness business maintains that you should accept. It doesn't make any difference whether you're 21 or 61 or whether you're in shape or not.

Regardless of what your identity is, I guarantee that you can change your body into anything you want.

Anyway, would you like my assistance? On the other hand, you replied "Yes!" you've taken the next step, not a stage, toward your objectives to turn into a less fatty, more solid you. Your excursion to a definitive female body starts when you go to the following page.

Chapter 1

What is your wellness why's

Finding and knowing your wellness for what reason is one of the most impressive mentality devices you consolidate toward the beginning of your wellness process.

This ties in intently and ought to be a piece of wellness objective setting, before you start, YOU want TO KNOW YOUR WHY.

Your wellness for what reason is the explanation you need to accomplish your objective. The most profound feelings and sentiments you have about yourself and your body. What you need to change and all the more significantly the explanation or justifications for why you need to roll out this improvement.

Everyone's reason will be different yet realizing yours will supercharge your objectives and put you in the best spot to crush through your usual ranges of familiarity.

You want to know precisely why and what you need to change before you can begin to transform it!

To make this as the need might arise to supercharge it. You want to burrow down somewhere inside yourself. Past all the shallow bs and hesitant responses and find out for yourself why you need this more than anything else.

You should be credible and 100 percent genuine for yourself. You thought of this objective for an explanation and just you know why that is.

Dig Profound To Track Down Your Why!

Now and again recognizing for what reason can raise feelings, might be covered way down inside your subliminal quality.

You might have made hindrances preventing it from rising to the top.

Regardless of how hard it is you want to burrow down, continue to wonder why, and for what reason would you like to accomplish these objectives. what is rousing you?

The uplifting news is the more feeling you can join to your why the better, the greater the inspiration, and the more impressive it becomes.

For what reason is Your Inspiration

Numerous clients tell me that I rouse them, I'm their inspiration and without me, they couldn't do it all alone. To be straightforward this isn't something I welcome and like.

I accept that inspiration is something you have or you don't have it's something you can be given or purchase.

As a fitness coach responsibility is what I give, an everyday practice and firm direction while you lose center. If you need inspiration, you are making this excursion a daunting struggle for the two of us, and the possibilities of you remaining on track to accomplish your objectives are thin.

One of the principal explanations behind lacking inspiration isn't recognizing and monitoring your why. Can we just be real if you don't have the foggiest idea why you are accomplishing something why might you continue to do it, particularly when it is as trying. as changing your everyday practice and your body?

For what reason is the explanation you will meaningfully have an impact on how you eat, the explanation you need to better yourself? It's the explanation you wake in the first part of the day, what gets you to the exercise centre, it is your inspiration and it empowers you to propel yourself more than you have at any point finished.

I can't track down your why for you. You need to do that for yourself. '

Reasons You Are Not Inspired to Change

I simply need to get some margin to specify a few different reasons which I feel might be the explanation or reasons you need inspiration.

1. You don't have the foggiest idea about your why.
2. You made your objective to satisfy another person or because you think it is what others would like.
3. You are searching for something to do because you are exhausted.
4. You need the outcomes yet you would rather not do any of the work it takes to accomplish them.
5. You were not ready for how much work you wanted to do.
6. You come up with too many reasons.
7. You are not ready to commit to how much time is expected to roll out the improvement.
8. Your idea that recruiting a mentor ensured results.

Here are only 8 focuses that I see consistently.

These are all mentality characteristics and are the reason in the body change pyramid I suggest guaranteeing you have serious areas of strength for a base before you start. A decent fitness coach/mentor ought to have the option to deal with your assumptions and provide you with a thought of what is expected before you start.

Tracking down Your Weight reduction Why
So how would you track down your wellness/weight reduction?
To distinguish your wellness I suggest having the Increasing present expectations objective setting layouts before you.
Sit in some place where you are distant from everyone else, have total quietness and ponder internally what are your objectives and for what reason would you like to accomplish them.
To find you're the reason you in a real sense continue to ask yourself for what reason and when you answer that why ask once more.

For instance:
*"I need to lose 3 stone of weight and drop my muscle versus fat ratio to 16%"
*WHY?
*Since my primary care physician has encouraged me to lose 3 stone and I accept that is a sound fat rate" (Outside impact)

*For what reason would I like to accomplish this objective?
"Since unexpectedly I have been told I am beefy beyond belief, I realised I was overweight yet never envisioned it was so awful"
*For what reason is this significant? how does this cause you to feel?"I do feel bad, I feel frustrated, I feel stunned, I feel terrified, I feel stressed, I feel miserable yet I not entirely set in stone to change this"
*For what reason are you so resolved now?"Because I am so near diabetes and other perilous ailments"

Continue to bore down till you track down sufficient fuel to keep your energy and fire consuming until your objectives are accomplished.

Do this for every objective.

*Recall the more reasons, feelings, and enthusiasm you can join to this the more remarkable it becomes

Record Your Wellness Why

Compose Everything DOWN!!

As you are boring down and refreshing your objectives, record your why, every one of the reasons that emerged as you drill down, and record the feelings and outcomes on the chance that you don't act now.

You need to lay out the greatest picture for yourself as could be expected and have the option to see it initially.

Utilise the free worksheet connected toward the finish of this blog.

Envision Your Why

This follows on from the last point, the most vital phase in imagining your reason is getting it on paper.

By recording it you are tracking down it, thinking it, saying it, composing it, seeing it, and pursuing it this cycle is solidifying it in your cerebrum.

As you will see on the entirety of my worksheets I inspire you to sign the base. For what reason do I do this as you are the main individual understanding it? This is another significant step that is modifying your psyche for progress.

Consider it agreeing with yourself, the substance you have composed is the thing you will do and by marking it you are pronouncing to yourself without help from anyone else that the work will be finished! At the point when you have gotten done and you have recorded everything on paper and marked you will put this somewhere you can see it regularly as well as someplace you approach it when you want.

Utilise these sheets as your inspirations while you lose concentration or feel deterred take a gander at these sheets, read them, and know why and recall the excursion you are on, why you began, and where you are focused on winding up.

As You Change So Does Your Why

Wellness ventures are something astonishing if you can remain on the way to progress.

Consistently I see clients changing before my eyes in actual appearance as well as in strength, wellness, well-being, certainty, self-discipline, and inspiration. As you change so too could your why and this is balance this is the ticket. Yet, remember your reason is important for the explanation you made so far so as you and your objectives change, update and revise your why.

Print off new layouts and worksheets and revamp them as the old ones have been vanquished and you have new objectives pushing ahead.

It is an incredibly strong outlook instrument to accomplish an objective and in this manner, your why changes, glance back at where you fired then tear it up and make fresh out of the plastic new objectives to accomplish things you never felt conceivable toward the beginning.

Chapter 2

The secret obstruction to accomplishing your well-being and wellness

Accomplishing your wellness objectives and adhering to a given activity routine is rarely simple. All things considered, there are a great deal of deterrents and obstructions like time, fatigue, wounds, examination, fearlessness, sluggishness, and so on.

In any case, these constraints can be crushed without any problem. In this way, whether you have laid out an objective to attempt another game, get in shape, or adhere to a wellness schedule, don't allow these obstructions to hold you up. Here we discuss what steps you can take to defeat normal deterrents and accomplish your wellness objectives.

Need more Chance To Exercise

Setting adequate time for practising can continuously be a test. With a smidgen of exertion and imagination, we can defeat this snag. If you need more time for a full exercise, you can do more limited eruptions of activity. Attempt to Crush in short strolls over the day. 'Drive less, walk more' ought to be the proverb of a bustling individual who needs to remain fit. It is said that life occurs in the night. In this way, get up only 30 minutes sooner than normal toward the beginning of the day and steadily increment if necessary. You can likewise redo your end-of-the-week fun by making it more exercise-situated. Transform your Sunday early show into a bicycle ride or journeying meeting. Along these lines, tomfoolery, and exercises can remain closely connected.

Practice Is Exhausting

It is completely normal to feel exhausted from a dull everyday practice. It is the equivalent with regards to working out too. Be that as it may, you can make practising more tomfoolery by adjusting your activity system. Guarantee that you incorporate exercises that you appreciate in your exercise. Additionally, shift the daily practice by pivoting among various exercises. Strolling, swimming, and cycling are the most ideal decisions for the equivalent. The more, the merrier. You can unite and practise with companions or colleagues. This way you will partake in the consolation and kinship. Likewise, keep your choices open by investigating new abilities.

Injury

Wounds can cause hopelessness, outrage, and even bitterness. Thus, to recuperate from wounds, you want to recognize the sentiments and foster an arrangement in a like manner. This recuperation period can likewise be pursued as an open door for you to draft new objectives. As opposed to feeling frail or feeble, you ought to enable yourself by tolerating what is going on. It means a lot to quickly return with another arrangement and it is basic to have an uplifting perspective. Having the appropriate spotlight on momentary accomplishments while you are harmed is likewise significant. You can take part in exercises that work for other muscle gatherings. This way you will remain connected with and dynamic. Likewise, guarantee that positive impact encompasses you. Rehearses like positive perception, contemplation, and hypnotherapy are helpful while recuperating a physical issue.

Sluggish To Exercise

On the off chance that taking a morning run makes you exhausted or drained, then track down different plans to remain fit. Ensure that you set reasonable assumptions. Assuming your objectives are excessively high, you might surrender without making a good attempt. Start with a stroll around your block. Ensure that you work with your temperament as opposed to against it. Plan exercises for the times you feel lively. This way you won't feel sluggish. Likewise, Timetable your exercises like you plan a pivotal arrangement. Along these lines, you won't feel that activities are discretionary.

Examination

The universe of games is extremely cutthroat. In this way, the examination may be unavoidable. In any case, estimating an individual's singular headway and making examinations are two various things. Making examinations with someone else could instigate sensations of dissatisfaction and insufficiency. However, estimating one's advancement will give trust, give space to development, and extend your fantasies. Self-assessment and objective setting are urgent for accomplishment. The most effective way to accomplish your objective is by laying out little objectives and changing over examinations into motivation.

The greater part of us know all about the most well-known obstruction to an ordinary actual work routine - - the absence of time. Work, family commitments, and different real factors of day-to-day existence frequently hinder our best expectations to be more dynamic. Numerous extra obstructions fluctuate by the individual and life situation.

On the off chance that you're focused on an actual work program and defining objectives for yourself, it's useful to initially recognize your obstructions. By investigating and creating strategies ahead of time, you'll have better achievement in beating them.

Here are a portion of the more normal boundaries and answers for conquering them:

1. Barrier: Absence of time

Arrangements: Screen your exercises for multi-week and distinguish somewhere around three, 30-minute spaces you could use for active work. Select exercises that you can squeeze into your home or work routine so you're not throwing away life on transportation to one more set to achieve them. Strolling in your area, climbing steps at your office, or practising while you sit in front of the television are great choices.

2. Barrier: Loved ones don't share your advantage in actual work

Arrangements: Make sense of your wellness or potential well-being improvement objectives to loved ones and request their help. Welcome companions to take part in active work with you. Join a nearby YMCA or strolling club to track down individuals with comparative objectives to offer help.

3. Barrier: Absence of inspiration as well as energy

Arrangements: Plan. Plan actual work for explicit times/days and "check" it off your rundown or schedule each time you complete it. Figure out what season of day you feel more vivacious and attempt to squeeze movement into that period. Join an activity gathering or class and look for others in the gathering to assist with propelling you and keep you responsible for joining in.

4. Barrier: Absence of assets/hardware

Arrangements: Select exercises that require negligible offices or hardware, like strolling, running, working out with rope, or working out. Distinguish reasonable, helpful assets locally, for example, parks and entertainment programs, worksite wellbeing gatherings, strolling clubs, and so on.

5. Barrier: Family providing care commitments
Arrangements: Exercise with your children - - take a walk together, play tag or other running match-ups, or get a vigorous dance or exercise tape for youngsters. You can hang out, possess the children, and guarantee they're getting the everyday actual work they need to remain solid. If you have a particular class, you like to join in, take a stab at exchanging watching with a neighbour.

6. Barrier: Continuous work or recreation travel
Arrangements: Join a YMCA or YWCA and get some information about proportional enrollments that permit admittance to offices in different urban communities. Pack a leap rope and opposition groups in your gear. Book inns that have a pool or potentially wellness rooms.

Chapter 3

Many people have barely any familiarity with well-being, nourishment, and wellness

We are living in a brilliant time of innovation and comfort. Measurably, a greater number of us have more cash and more open doors than at any time in recent memory. Regardless of that open door, a greater amount of us are likewise unhealthier than at any time in recent memory.

The world is held in a significant weight emergency, emotional wellness conditions are on the ascent and as per the World Wellbeing Association, more than 300 million individuals overall are presently living with despondency. These are dynamic issues that need dynamic arrangements to work on the general status of our well-being.

More significant still, it merits calling attention to the fact that no two individuals are similar. That implies what works for certain individuals to accomplish better well-being may not work for everybody. Yet, there are normal focuses that everyone ought to remember while attempting to work on their well-being.

If you're searching for new manners by which to work on your well-being (mental, physical, or a blend of the two), we've gathered together five key realities for you to remember on your excursion.

1. Avoidance Is The Best Treatment

Nowadays, by far most of us just head to a specialist to take care of an issue.

When we at last look for clinical help, we spend much of the time managing persistent issues that can be quite difficult to tackle. You've heard it said multiple times, "Counteraction is the best medication," and even "no medication can beat a healthy lifestyle." In The End, our grandparents understood what they were referring to!

We should investigate heftiness for instance. Being overweight can cause an extensive variety of medical conditions, including:

Diabetes

Outer muscle problems

Diseases
Cardiovascular infections

As per the WHO, a singular's possibility of becoming overweight and fostering these circumstances can be diminished by simplifying a couple of life changes like restricting our admission of greasy food sources or handled sugars and expanding utilisation of products of the soil.

These are the basic way of life changes that can forestall serious medical issues - so don't hold on until you have some weird side effects or begin to feel dreadful to make a beeline for the specialist and request help. Figure out how you can forestall future issues and make a move today.

2. You Want To Get More Rest

We as a whole carry on with occupied lives, and frequently we wind up taking on too much work to get by or keep up with any kind of public activity. Be that as it may, you can't do quite a bit of anything while you're running on empty, so to work on your well-being, ensure you're getting sufficient rest.

As per the CDC, 35% of grown-ups in the US log under seven hours of rest an evening. Yet, grown-ups who are somewhere in the range of 18 and 60 years of age require over seven hours of rest each night to appropriately work the next day - and assuming that you're more than 60, it's prescribed you get as long as nine hours out of every evening. Assuming you believe that enough energy should perform at work, practice, and keep up with sound connections, you must ensure you're dozing enough. This is one of the most critical, yet neglected bits of this riddle!

3. Watch What You Eat

At the point when we're in a rush, we frequently follow the easy way out to what we will eat as opposed to pausing and thinking about what we're going to ingest. Yet, truly, food is medication - so you must mull over what's in your food and plan your feasts.

What precisely does a fair eating routine focusing on a sound weight involve? As indicated by the CDC, your eating regimen ought to:

Focus on foods grown from the ground
Underscore entire grains and sans-fat milk
Be low in immersed fats
Remain inside your day-to-day calorie needs

Past contributions your body the fuel it necessitates to continue onward, and quality and good food additionally can help you loosen up and foster your connections to work on psychological wellness. Food can be social, and you ought to appreciate it.

4. You Want To Dial Back

At the point when you're centred around getting out there, reaching out, and making every moment count, you might be enticed to ride out fatigue. Help yourself out and don't.

While you're feeling tired, you want to dial back. Advise yourself that it's OK to pause and calmly inhale - whether you're at home, work, or elsewhere. Rest is a fundamental piece of genuine efficiency. On the off chance that you must be regimental about it, you could take what some have named a "computerised time of rest," time every day or week in which you're focused on keeping away from screens, quit browsing messages, and get the hell off of web-based entertainment.

Not only will this work on your emotional wellness, but it can affect your actual capacity to adapt to anything your day tosses at you.

5. You Ought to work out Each Day

OK, this could sound like a piece two-faced after advising you to dial back and enjoy some time off however hold on for us. As indicated by the CDC, just 23% of Americans practise enough. Latency can prompt a wide range of issues, and you would rather not be THAT measurement!

In any case, in all honesty, the everyday workout you want is a ton more straightforward than you could suspect. We're not talking long-distance races here. Direction from the Mayo Facility suggests that all grown-ups ought to hold back nothing objective of something like 30 minutes of moderate actual work every day.

What's moderate? You could attempt a lively walk, swimming, or trimming the grass. On the other hand, on the off chance that you're prepared to take your activity to a higher level, you could have a go at running, or far better: a workout schedule like combative techniques!

By practising every day, you'll keep up with great actual well-being that will assist with helping your emotional well-being, as well. That is the reason day-to-day practice is one of the main taking care of oneself practises you can lock in.

Chapter 4

The most effective method to eat good food while you assemble the body you need

Attempt to eat less soaked fat and pick food sources that contain unsaturated fats all things being equal, like vegetable oils and spreads, slick fish, and avocados. For a better decision, utilize a limited quantity of vegetable or olive oil, or decrease.

Eating an even eating regimen can assist you with getting the calories and supplements you want to fuel your everyday exercises, including standard activity.

With regards to eating food sources to fuel your activity execution, it's not generally so basic as picking vegetables over doughnuts. You want to eat the ideal sorts of food at the perfect times.

Your most memorable dinner of the day is a significant one.

Having breakfast consistently has been connected to a lower hazard of heftiness, diabetes, and coronary illness. Beginning your day with a quality feast can assist with renewing your glucose, which your body needs to drive your muscles and cerebrum.

Having a sound breakfast is particularly significant on days when exercise is on your plan. Skipping breakfast can leave you feeling dizzy or lazy while you're working out.

Picking the right sort of breakfast is essential. Such a large number of individuals depend on basic starches to begin their day.

A plain white bagel or donut won't keep you feeling full for a long time.

In correlation, a fibre- and protein-rich breakfast might fight off cravings for food for longer and give you the energy you want to push your activity along.

Follow these methods to have a sound breakfast:
Instead of eating sugar-loaded cereals produced using refined grains, try oats, oat wheat, or other entire-grain cereals that are high in fibre. Then, toss in some protein, like milk, yoghurt, or chopped nuts. If you're making hotcakes or waffles, supplant a portion of the regular baking flour with entire grain choices. Then, mix some curds into the batter. If you are inclined toward toast, pick entire-grain bread. Then, at that point, match it with an egg, peanut butter, or another protein source.

Rely on the right carbs
Because of the low-carb craze slims down, starches have gotten negative criticism. In any case, sugars are your body's principal wellspring of energy. As indicated by the Mayo Facility, around 45 to 65 percent of your all-out day-to-day calories ought to come from sugars. This is particularly evident on the off chance that you work out.
Consuming the right sort of starches is significant. Many individuals depend on the basic carbs tracked

down in desserts and handled food varieties. All things being equal, you ought to zero in on eating the complex carbs tracked down in entire grains, natural products, vegetables, and beans.

Entire grains have more resilience than refined grains since you digest them all the more leisurely.

They can assist you with feeling full for longer and fuel your body over the day. They can likewise assist with balancing out your glucose levels.

At long last, these quality grains have the nutrients and minerals you want to keep your body running at its ideal.

Nourishment is significant for wellness

Eating an even eating routine can assist you with getting the calories and supplements you want to fuel your everyday exercises, including standard activity.

With regards to eating food sources to fuel your activity execution, it's not quite as straightforward as picking vegetables over doughnuts. You want to eat the ideal sorts of food at the perfect times.

Find out about the significance of sound morning meals, exercise tidbits, and feast plans.

Start very strong

Your most memorable dinner of the day is a significant one.

As per an article distributed in Harvard Wellbeing Letter, having breakfast routinely has been connected to a lower chance of corpulence, diabetes, and coronary illness. Beginning your day with a good dinner can assist with recharging your glucose, which your body needs to drive your muscles and mind.

Having a sound breakfast is particularly significant on days when exercise is on your plan. Missing breakfast can leave you feeling dazed or lazy while you're working out.

Picking the right sort of breakfast is pivotal. An excessive number of individuals depend on basic carbs to begin their day.

A plain white bagel or donut won't keep you feeling full for a long time.

In the examination, a fibre-and protein-rich breakfast might fight off food cravings for longer and give the energy you want to make a big difference in your activity.

Pack protein into your tidbits and feasts

Protein is expected to assist with keeping your body developing, kept up with, and fixed. For instance, red platelets bite the dust after around 120 days.

Protein is likewise fundamental for building and fixing muscles, assisting you with partaking in the advantages of your exercise. It tends to be a wellspring of energy when carbs are hard to find, however, it's anything but a significant wellspring of fuel during exercise.

Grown-ups need to eat around 0.8 grams of protein each day for each kilogram of their body weight, reports Harvard Wellbeing Site. That is equivalent to around 0.36 grams of protein for each pound of body weight. Exercisers and more established grown-ups may require significantly more.

Protein can emerge out of:
*poultry, like chicken and turkey
*red meat, like hamburger and sheep
*fish, like salmon and fish
*dairy, like milk and yoghourt
*vegetables, like beans and lentils
*Eggs

For the best choices, pick lean proteins that are low in soaked and trans fats. Limit how much red meat and handled meats that you eat.

Help your leafy foods admission

Products of the soil are rich wellsprings of regular fibre, nutrients, minerals, and different mixtures that your body needs to appropriately work. They're low in calories and fat.

Intend to fill a portion of your plate with foods grown from the ground at each dinner, suggests the US Division of Farming.

Attempt to "eat the rainbow" by picking foods grown from the ground of various varieties. This will assist you with partaking in the full scope of nutrients, minerals, and cancer prevention agents that the produce path brings to the table.

Each time you go to the supermarket, consider picking another natural product or vegetable to attempt. For snacks, keep dried natural products in your exercise sack and crude veggies in the ice chest.

Pick solid fats

Unsaturated fats might assist with lessening aggravation and give calories.

While fat is an essential fuel for high-impact workouts, we have a bounty put away in the body to fuel even the longest exercises. Be that as it may, getting solid unsaturated fats assists with giving fundamental unsaturated fats and calories to keep you moving.

Solid choices include:
nuts
seeds
avocados
olives
oils, like olive oil

Fuel up before working out
With regards to powering up last or after an exercise, it's essential to accomplish the right equilibrium of carbs and protein. Pre-exercise tidbits that combine carbs with protein can cause you to feel more empowered than unhealthy foods produced using basic sugars and bunches of fat.
Consider loading your exercise sack and fridge with a portion of these straightforward bites:

Bananas

Bananas are brimming with potassium and magnesium, which are significant supplements to get consistently. Eating a banana can assist with recharging these minerals while giving regular sugars to fuel your exercise. For added protein, partake in your banana with a serving of peanut butter.

Berries, grapes, and oranges
These natural products are brimming with nutrients, minerals, and water. They're kind to your digestive organs, provide you with a speedy increase in energy, and assist you with remaining hydrated. Think about matching them with a serving of yogurt for protein.

Nuts
Nuts are an extraordinary wellspring of heart-sound fats and give protein and fundamental supplements. They can give you a wellspring of supported energy for your exercise.
Match them with new or dried natural products for a solid portion of carbs. Notwithstanding, test these choices to perceive how they settle. High-fat food

varieties can slow absorption, and they might cause food to sit in your stomach excessively lengthy assuming your exercise is coming up rapidly.

Nut margarine
Numerous supermarkets convey single-serving parcels of peanut butter that don't need refrigeration and can be effectively put away in a duffel bag. For a scrumptious protein-carb combo, you can spread peanut butter on:
*an apple
*a banana
*entire grain wafers
*a cut of entire-grain bread

If you could do without peanut butter, attempt almond spread, soy margarine, or other protein-rich options.

Try not to cut an excessive number of calories
If you're attempting to get in shape or tone your body, you might be enticed to cut a lot of calories from your feasts. Cutting calories is a vital piece of weight reduction, however, it's feasible to go excessively far.

Weight reduction diets ought to never leave you feeling depleted or sick. Those are signs that you're not getting the calories you want for good well-being and wellness.

As indicated by the Public Heart, Lung, and Blood Organization, an eating routine containing 1,200 to 1,500 day-to-day calories is reasonable for most ladies who are attempting to securely get in shape. An eating routine with 1,500 to 1,800 every day calories is fitting for most men who are attempting to shed overabundance pounds.

To get thinner while getting fit, you might have to eat more calories. Converse with your PCP or a dietitian to figure out the number of calories you need to help your way of life and wellness objectives.

Balance is critical

As you subside into a functioning way of life, you'll presumably find which food varieties give you the most energy and which have adverse consequences. The key is figuring out how to pay attention to your body and offsetting what feels right with what you want.

Follow these tips:

*Intend to make breakfast a piece of your everyday practice.

*Pick complex carbs, lean protein sources, solid fats, and a wide assortment of foods grown from the ground.

*Stock your ice chest and a duffel bag with sound exercise snacks.

The right equilibrium of sugars, protein, and different supplements can assist with powering your workout daily practice.

Chapter 5

The most effective method to forestall exercise wounds

Working out at home enjoys numerous benefits. It's helpful, and cost-productive, you approach the gear you want constantly and it likewise can make a decent holding action with your friends and family. In any case, exercise wounds can happen whenever, even at home, particularly while you're lifting loads or doing an extreme focus routine with an ill-advised stance and structure. Certain individuals additionally watch out for exercise exorbitantly at home which might destroy muscles as well as bother existing wounds or conditions, for example, joint or knee torment.

Before we examine far to forestall encountering wounds, we should initially bring a glance at the normal back home exercise wounds underneath:

7 Normal Home Exercise Wounds

1. Sprains or wounds to tendons because of unplanned turns

2. Muscle or ligament wounds from not heating up

3. Tendinitis or irritation of a ligament because of abuse

4. Lower back torment due to lifting with ill-advised structure

5. Hip or knee torment because of unnecessary exercises

6. Hamstring force brought about by speedy, startling developments

7. Shoulder impingement because of extreme above activities with inappropriate behaviour

The most effective method to Forestall Home Exercise Wounds
Here are far to forestall encountering the normal home exercise wounds.
1. Warm up and chill off.
Extending, energetic strolling and additional running setup before working out can assist with setting up your muscles and your pulse for your daily schedule, forestall strain, and try not to inhale issues. Doing these after exercise can likewise assist with chilling your body off and gradually assist your heart with rating full recovery.

2. Practise appropriate structure and stance.
Keeping up with great structure and stance can assist you with really practising the right muscles as well as forestall joint, shoulder, and back torment.

3. Wear a decent set of shoes with curved support.
Long exercises and various redundancies can put weight on your joints and feet, so make certain to wear a decent set of shoes to stay away from any opportunity of irritation or injury. On the off chance

that you favour doing high-affect works, putting resources into a couple of running shoes with great cushioning would be ideal.

4. Use mats to forestall joint agony and slipping mishaps.
It's not prudent to figure out a floor covering, hardwood, concrete, or even carpets and towels as they can prompt slipping mishaps. The most ideal decision is a thick activity or yoga mat, particularly when your exercise includes bounces, boards, and different activities that expect you to sit down.

5. Try not to propel yourself excessively hard.
It is important to Pay attention to your body. On the off chance that you feel like you can't take another set, then, at that point, pause and begin chilling off following a couple of moments. Try not to propel yourself past your breaking point to stay away from ligament irritation, muscle tears, injuries, and joint agony.

6. Allow your body to recuperate.
Your muscles expect time to recuperate. Make sure to get sufficient rest, eat sufficient protein, and timetable your exercises such that you can in any

case rest, particularly assuming you come from a stationary way of life and have begun working out as of late.

Last Contemplations

If you experience any of these home exercise wounds, if it's not too much trouble, counsel a specialist straightaway to forestall more prominent well-being gambles from here on out. For perilous crises like cracks and weighty dying, if it's not too much trouble, call 911. Remain safe!

Chapter 6

10 Normal Weight Reduction Legends, Busted

Separate reality from fiction about a portion of the broadly acknowledged confusion around slimming down and weight reduction.

Weight reduction can be a muddled, confounding, and profound cycle, with clashing guidance coming from each course. Perhaps your folks or companions have affected your dietary patterns through unsafe remarks — regardless of how good-natured. Or then again you're clutching now-exposed lessons from secondary school wellbeing class. For the vast majority, virtual entertainment patterns (taking a gander at you, "What I eat in a day" pattern) are raising questions about the things we're eating.

It's critical to comprehend that the interaction is different for everybody and to isolate reality from fiction. So we should get into probably the most widely recognized legends about shedding pounds and the reality behind them.

1. Myth: Skipping dinners is an effective method for getting more fit rapidly.

Reality: Skipping feasts can dial back your digestion and make weight reduction harder — among other unsafe impacts.

Eating ordinary feasts assists you with controlling your digestion and provides your body with a reliable inventory of supplements — fundamental for keeping a sound load over the long run. Also, skipping feasts can prompt gorging or revelling in undesirable snacks later on, which could make you put on weight. Eating more modest, more continuous dinners over the day can assist you with remaining focused and keeping away from food cravings.

Keep in mind that eating ordinary feasts with heaps of nutritious food sources like organic products, vegetables, lean proteins, and complex starches will give you the energy and centre you want to keep on settling on better conclusions about the food varieties you're eating. It's a cycle! Eating nutritious feasts consistently can assist you with keeping a sound weight and feeling your best.

2. Myth: having dinner late causes weight gain.

Reality: Late-evening eating won't make you put on weight — as long as you remember a couple of things.

"It is a legend," says dietician Sinan Ozyemisci, MS, RDN. "Eating late around evening time is not an immediate reason for weight gain." In any case, he takes note of that similarly as with everything, there are provisos. For example, on the off chance that you've proactively met your carbohydrate content objective for the afternoon, eating late around evening time prompts overconsumption.

"On the other hand, on the off chance that we sit before the television, there's in many cases no piece control," says Sinan. "On the off chance that I'm at a film, I'm not including the number of bits of popcorn that I'm eating all through that film. I'm simply eating that extra-large popcorn. I think segment control sort of vacates the premises when it's later in the day."

One more element to consider is what eating late in the evening time could mean for your rest. Eating just before bed can mean nodding off and feeling awkward for some, whether that is because of feeling full or consuming a great deal of sugar that keeps you from resting sufficiently. "The next day, you will be working on less rest, which is going to lead your body to maintain that more calories all together should work at an ideal level" makes sense Sinan.

In this manner, it's essential to consider the kinds of food and the bits you eat. Eating late around evening time is fine for however long you're eating a fair eating regimen, so don't let the legend of late-evening eating and weight gain hold you back from partaking in a solid tidbit or dinner. With careful piece control and nutritious food decisions, you can partake in your number one late-night treat with next to no coercion.

3. Myth: Doing lots of cardio will assist you with consuming fat all the more rapidly.
Reality: Cardio alone is much of the time adequate not to get fitter.
It's essential to join cardio with strength preparation and a solid eating regimen. Together, these three parts can assist you with making a viable weight reduction plan.
While cardio can assist with supporting your digestion and consuming calories, strength-preparing practices are astounding for weight reduction since they require the body to use more energy (otherwise known as consuming more

calories). So, you acquire bulk and lose more weight. A sound eating regimen gives the fuel your body needs to stay aware of your workout daily schedule. Working out routinely, eating adjusted feasts, and monitoring your calorie admission are key parts of a fruitful weight reduction plan. Recall that consistency is critical — the more you keep focused, the improved outcomes you'll find over the long haul.

4. Myth: Drinking water will assist you with getting thinner.
Reality: This is valid! Sort of.
Water is not a supernatural serum that will lead you to shed pounds. All things considered, drinking water can assist with weight reduction when part of a generally speaking better way of life. For example, drinking a lot of water throughout the morning was found to stifle hunger in those classified as "would be expected weight," yet didn't recognizably affect those categorised as overweight or fat.
One demonstrated truth, in any case, is that remaining hydrated makes practice simpler, assisting you with working out longer and at higher forces. Who would rather not make indisputably the most out of every exercise?

5. Myth: Eating under 1,000 calories each day will assist you with getting more fit.

Reality: Eating too many calories can make it harder for you to get in shape over the long haul.

Eating too many calories can prompt weakness, desires, and gorging, and it can dial back your digestion. Eating a solid, offset diet with the right number of calories is critical to effective weight reduction. Furthermore, it's critical to ensure you get an adequate number of nutrients and minerals in your eating routine, which can be no picnic for a low-calorie diet.

Eating fewer calories than your body needs to fuel fundamental capabilities can likewise cause other medical problems and influence each organ framework in the body. Your body will begin to separate its tissues, and muscles are the principal target. This incorporates your heart, which can begin to respond by bringing down your pulse and circulatory strain and expanding your gamble for cardiovascular breakdown after some time. Different outcomes include:

Feeling frail, tired, or bad-tempered Having dry, dull skin and fragile hair, or encountering hair loss

Getting debilitated on a more regular basis and more severely being able to get warm

One choice is to eat five little feasts a day, with every dinner having somewhere in the range of 300 and 500 calories. This will assist with keeping your energy steps up while ensuring you don't go over your calorie limit for the afternoon. This is only an overall suggestion, and we as a whole have different dietary requirements.

It's really smart to gain proficiency with your exceptional metabolic rate and caloric admission proposals — which is precisely the thing the Evolt body piece scanner does. Also, the uplifting news is that each AF rec centre has an Evolt scanner that can investigate your exceptional body with more than 40 unique sorts of estimations. Ask your Mentor or rec centre staff about setting up an arrangement to get the simple 60-second sweep.

6. Myth: Eating servings of mixed greens consistently will prompt weight reduction.

Reality: Mixed greens are an extraordinary method for getting in loads of supplements, yet they will not be guaranteed to prompt weight reduction.

Assuming you're adding unhealthy garnishes like cheddar, rich dressing, and bread garnishes, your serving of mixed greens could be counterproductive to your weight reduction endeavours. To ensure your plates of mixed greens are helping and not thwarting your objectives, settle on sound garnishes like barbecued chicken, nuts, seeds, or avocado.

One more worry with eating just plates of mixed greens is that you'll deny yourself of the food varieties you love, which frequently prompts unhealthy food desires. Part of keeping a durable relationship with smart dieting is revealing from time to time!

7. Myth: Eating greasy food sources will make you fat.

Reality: Practising good eating habits with some restraint won't prompt weight gain.

There's a misguided judgement that food varieties marked as "low fat" or "diminished fat" are consistently a better decision, yet truly, there are totally solid fats — and your body depends on them. Diets tracked down in olive oil, nuts, and fish can assist you with feeling full for longer and give fundamental unsaturated fats that your body needs to work.

It's essential to be aware of part sizes and cut unfortunate trans and soaked fats. Eating an excess of unfortunate fat can prompt weight gain. Take a stab at balance by remembering a lot of foods grown from the ground for your eating regimen too.

8. Myth: Carbs are awful for you.
Reality: Sugars are a significant piece of a fair eating regimen.
We've all heard it: Carbs are awful. Trend consumes fewer calories and deceiving titles drill this into our heads since early on. This is old information. Carbs are your body's favoured wellspring of energy (which is uplifting news given that cutting carbs from your eating routine is an unreasonable way to deal with weight reduction).

Entire grains like oats, quinoa, and earthy-coloured rice are intricate sugars that can give your body energy and fundamental nutrients and minerals.

Eating these sound carbs with some restraint can assist your body with keeping a solid weight, further develop processing, and even lower your gamble for constant illnesses. By staying away from handled food varieties with added sugars and deciding on supplements with thick entire grains, you can guarantee that carbs are a helpful and fundamental piece of your eating routine.

9. Myth: Better food varieties are more costly.

Reality: It is feasible to eat soundly on a careful spending plan, yet it might require some work, arranging, and innovativeness.

Indeed, entire or insignificantly handled food varieties like natural products, vegetables, entire grains, and incline proteins can be more costly than their handled partners. A few investigations have shown that better food sources will generally be more costly than their undesirable partners. In 2013, for example, the Harvard School of General Well Being found that it costs a normal $1.50 more each day to steadily eat.

In any case, the concentrate just took a gander at the expense per calorie, as opposed to the expense per serving. It analysed the expense of 200 calories worth of cake to 200 calories worth of broccoli. The piece of cake would include calories a whole lot faster than the broccoli. Thus, rather than zeroing in on calories alone, ensure you.

There are other amazing ways of ensuring good dieting is more reasonable, including:

1. Buy durable food sources in mass. There are lots of nutritious canned, frozen, and dry food sources that you can purchase in enormous amounts at a

lower cost — without the feeling of dread toward them turning sour. "I think canned beans are one of the No. 1 sources no matter how you look at it," says Sinan. "They're an incredible protein hotspot for our veggie lover and vegan populace, as well as the meat eaters." His other top picks include:

Quinoa
Oats
 Canned salmon
Canned chicken
Nuts
Dried natural products

2.Eat in. Feasting out is a genuine illustration of when it costs more to eat commonly less good food sources. Also, cooking for yourself implies knowing precisely the very thing fixings are in your feasts.

3. Plan. We know, it's quite difficult. However, it's a propensity that you CAN frame and the advantages are perfect. Arranging feasts and staple records early can assist you with setting aside cash by guaranteeing that you're just purchasing what you want for explicit recipes, instead of superfluously loading up on fixings.

While these tips can assist with having a major effect on how you approach good dieting, actually sometimes, better food decisions can be more costly. Be that as it may, we inquire: What's more critical to put resources into than your well-being?

10. Myth: All calories are equivalent.
Reality: The wellspring of calories influences how your body utilises them.
One calorie gives a similar measure of energy as the following, yet not all calories pack a similar punch with regards to the health benefits they convey — or how your body answers them. What makes them unique? The food source they come from. A few sources might give more valuable sustenance than others. For instance, 100 calories from sugars will be handled uniquely in contrast to 100 calories from fat.
Devouring unhealthy food varieties that are low in sustenance can prompt weight gain since they don't furnish your body with supported energy or significant wholesome parts.
Different calorie sources can likewise unexpectedly influence appetite and totality. Eating protein-rich food sources like meat, eggs, and nuts can cause you

to feel more full for longer than if you were eating carbs or fat alone.

So about calories, quality matters! It's critical to focus on the wellspring of calories while pursuing dietary choices. What makes the biggest difference is picking supplement-thick food sources that give a fair admission of macronutrients, micronutrients, and other valuable substances.

The reality is this: Weight reduction is a perplexing and individual interaction. There is no one-size-fits-all way to deal with weight reduction, and finding that employer and your lifestyle is significant. With the right direction and backing, you can effectively arrive at your objectives!

Chapter 7

The inward round of getting fit

The inward game

The ref gives you the ball. Crawling your foot up to the free-toss line, you eyeball the clock: only seconds left and your group is one point behind. Your mentor has that look; he's relying on you.

Taking a full breath, you're innervated by the steps, whistles, cheers, applause, air horns, and cowbells. It zaps you. You turn the ball in your grasp, fingering the line your palm knows best. One delicate squat, a lift, and a hand loosened up over the loop… Wash.

The score is tied. One more banked shot and it's yours. Your partners edge out space in the key, asserting safeguard.

Power shoots through you and, surprisingly, the reciting in the stands vanishes as the nearsighted perspective on the edge fills your cerebrum. You're in the zone and everything comes down to you. That subsequent shot clears the net perfectly and the group goes wild.

You figured out your perfect balance.

Therapists refer to this as "stream," your capacity to turn out to be so charmed in an action that your body goes on autopilot. You've most likely experienced it previously - the inclination that nothing can stop you, that you have this.

For this reason, we train, the regular high, being most inside our bodies, expecting a profit from what we put resources into the work. Regardless of the action you love, you request restitution. Furthermore, when you arrive at an objective, it powers your power and longing for more.

What Keeps You Preparing?

What keeps you preparing? New private records, rivalry, the test of another exercise, social help, shedding 50 pounds, or putting muscles on what used to be twiggy arms and legs?

You're now devoted to working it out, however, what happens when you're "off" your game?

Understanding your internal inspiration is foremost to long-term achievement. Inspiration can be either extraneous (the carrot draped out before you), or natural (got comfortable in your stomach, the assurance that you won't withdraw under any circumstance).

I feel that both are useful and either can be excessively outrageous.

Why Not Outer Inspirations As it were?

Exercises and diets are multitudinous. Specialists proliferate, each letting you know they have precisely the exact thing you're searching for. Letting a person or thing else be your normal inspiration can leave you baffled.

Assuming you pursue an endless flow of choices, searching for the "amazing fit," you could continuously be searching for your perfect balance.

Fostering a relationship with your characteristic inspiration expects you to get alone with yourself sufficiently long to know what "makes you tick." As a fitness coach, I observe that this is more hard for individuals.

It's not difficult to be misdirected by the possibility that our desires for well-being are sufficient to make us more grounded. In any case, what happens when you get worn out, your coach moves, or your exercise accomplice smothers his knee?

Realise what moves you when you're not ablaze. Me? I want one thing in life that I associate with my repressed monster. I need to decide that. I want a couple of things that I can do pretty well. I want something that I'm learning, a spot to investigate. What's more, beyond that, I want a healthy lifestyle — on the off chance that it doesn't fit within balance, I minimise the need, it is enjoyable to let it.

And You? Do You Have at least some Idea What Spurs You When You Need Outside Motivation?

*Calm Time - This can directly up suck for some individuals. Be that as it may, realising when to depressurize and when to push hard will assist with safeguarding you against losing force by and large when you experience a change throughout everyday life.

*Finding your "Rarrr" - As far as I might be concerned, this is the way to characteristic inspiration. I flourish with experience and force. Thoroughly consider the times you've been lost in an action, sure to the place of narcissism. No one could stop you.

*Limit Outward Compensations for a Period - What will you work for with next to no reward at all?

Search for things that would get you up at 5 am and fabricate a fair program around them!

*Personality - My meetings with clients begin something similar — "I need to get better, shed pounds, and tone up." The ideal image of their constitution and how I program them toward that will be remarkable for every client.

*Getting Genuine - The more seasoned we get, the more certain that we have profound or mental hang-ups remaining among us and what we need. The more you're alright with calling poo what it is, the less time you'll squander.

The ref gives you the ball. You anxiously take it from him and eye the clock. You're spooky, knowing that with just seconds left and somewhere around one, you have to possess this.

The group is alarming, and you wish that the commotion would stop so you could focus. The ball feels off-kilter in your grasp and you simply maintain that this second should pass. Teeth gritted, you hop excessively high, the ball failing against the backboard to a quiet quietness.

Everything comes down to you. Will you break or will you understand what carried you to this point?

Chapter 8

The straightforward rationale of determination and restraint

We as a whole wish we had more resolution, self-control, and restraint.

All things considered, ponder what we could do and all we could accomplish assuming we did.

A few specialists genuinely think expanding how we might interpret resolve and restraint might be brain research's best expectation in adding to human government assistance.

All things considered, the abundance of self-improvement guides at the air terminal recommends we as a whole need assistance to shape beneficial routines and be more focused as we pursue our objectives.

What Is Resolved? Its Importance and Definition
Neuroscience lets us know that the prefrontal piece of the mind simply behind our temple controls what we do. It guides what we pay attention to and think about and, surprisingly, the feelings we experience.
In this way, when we put things off, staring at the television as opposed to finishing the tax document, that is our prefrontal cortex at work.
But, this piece of the cerebrum is more than a solitary brought-together chief. It has three key regions, everyone assisting us with weighing up whether "I will," "I will not," or "I need" to follow through with something.
The left half of this cerebrum locale assists us with adhering to undertakings (I will)- in any event, exhausting ones-while the right side (I won't) prevents us from being diverted or yielding to enticement. At long last, in the centre, however, lower down in our prefrontal cortex, the cells fire to keep us roused and by our objectives (I need).
At times, on account of the continuous rivalry inside our minds, we fall flat. We don't have the self-

control to adhere to the eating regimen or get to the rec centre. At different times, we keep up with the drive to push on, regardless of different interests, enticements, and interruptions. Self-discipline is obvious in the last option.

Going ahead "anybody with some educational experience added to their repertoire realises that they can achieve more with a solid feeling of requirement and determination.

All in all, where does this leave us with our comprehension - its significance and definition?

Self-discipline is the capacity to oppose transient enticements to meet long-haul objectives.

We could characterise resolve and see its advantages as:

*Opposing momentary allurements and postponing satisfaction to accomplish long-haul objectives

*Abrogating undesirable considerations, sentiments, or motivations

*Answering coolly and serenely instead of acting too sincerely

*Cognizant, effortful guideline of oneself without help from anyone else

*A restricted asset that can be exhausted

Understanding resolve is fundamental to perceiving the reason why we act as we do and how we foster our flexibility.

For quite a while, clinicians considered resolving a restricted asset — known as the 'inner self-consumption hypothesis'

self-discipline is limited and very much like energy when muscles are exhausted can be spent. In his well-known 'treat' exploration, individuals who could oppose destroying their right (called deferred satisfaction) had a really difficult time controlling enticement later in different errands.

That's what the hypothesis recommends: assuming you set more than one personal development objective, you might draw on resolve saves, leaving you drained and flirting with disappointment.

What's more, if self-discipline is a restricted asset, we should utilise it carefully to accomplish long-haul objectives.

However, ongoing and disconnected mental examination and hypothesis propose there is certainly not a proper measure of determination. "Rather than considering self-control how much petrol is in a vehicle… consider it the vehicle's battery,"

With the right mentality and inspiration, we can 'claim' our restraint and resolve. Furthermore, this is upheld by information. Concentrates on showing that individuals are less inclined to stop an undertaking when told their purpose isn't fixed however limitless.

While building determination is difficult, brain science recommends that "a colossal piece of the arrangement is accepting that you can make it happen".

All in all, what happens when we do and don't finish things?

It appears to be that attitude is urgent. Understudies coming up to tests that were informed resolution was limitless, experienced less pressure, less awful states of mind, and could increase their determination. If we 'accept,' we have the stores accessible to handle the difficulties ahead, we increment our possibilities of future achievement.

Excellent Instances of Resolve

The accompanying three strong models feature the potential for self-control to change lives.

The main shows how it is possible to lose our solidarity of will and what it is meant for by the cerebrum's life structures. The second shows the worth of resolution in sports and the last shows the capability of beneficial routines to further develop business execution.

The inquisitive instance of Phineas Gage
While dealing with the railroads in 1848, quarter-century-old Phineas Gage experienced a horrendous mishap. An iron bar penetrated his skull at speed following a blast, dwelling itself in his prefrontal cortex. Even though he endured the head injury, he encountered outrageous changes to his character, language, knowledge, engine capabilities, and restraint.

Beforehand quiet, engaged, and intellectually solid, he was presently fretful and hasty. His companions portrayed him as done being Gage — he had lost his most respected characteristics, especially his self-discipline.

The harm to the piece of the mind we presently know is related to discretion implying that he no longer had the self-control to own undertakings as far as possible or to prevent himself from capitulating to enticement. He never completely recuperated.

A baseball legend
Kobe Bryant was an American b-ball player generally viewed as one of the flat-out best. He was known for areas of strength and assurance all through his b-ball vocation.
But, having joined a late spring ball camp at age 12, he didn't score a solitary point. He was prepared to abandon the ball, however, at that point, he read about how Michael Jordan was cut from his secondary school b-ball group and how it turned into his inspiration to outpace everybody around him.
The story motivated Kobe to emulate Jordan's example and turn into the hardest labourer in the sport of b-ball. He started appearing at the exercise centre at 5 am and holding off on leaving until 7 pm while in secondary school. He put himself through four hours of extraordinary exercise routines even on game days, played one-on-one games up to 100 focuses after training, and chipped away at his abilities with no other person or a ball to consummate his footwork.

Michael Jordan was a good example and motivation for Kobe, enormously impacting his self-control and inspiring him to accomplish his objectives.

Tragically, Kobe's life was stopped by a staggering helicopter crash in 2020 that killed him and his girl, yet he was to turn into a motivation for his fans, and his responsibility an example to every one of us.

Persevering for social liberties

Rosa Stops never envisioned that her transport process home would bring about her turning into a nonentity for the US social equality development.

But, on December 1, 1955, when she was captured for declining to surrender her seat for a white individual, it prompted a 381-day blacklist and a definitive cancelation of racial isolation on transports (Bredhoff, Wynell, and Potter, 1999).

Rosa Parks' solidarity of will made one little demonstration of rebellion that was important for something that changed history and her being referred to by the US Congress as "the principal woman of social liberties

Making beneficial routines to help resolve

James Clear discusses the significance of good methodologies in his book "Nuclear Propensities" and offers the accompanying illustration of how they can drive determination.

At the point when Trent Dyrsmid started his position at a bank in 1993, he was youthful and unpracticed - so nobody anticipated much from him. But, he shaped a strong propensity that supported his responsibility and determination.

He began every day with two containers: one with 120 paper cuts and the other void. Each time he settled on a deal decision, he moved one paperclip from the full container to the unfilled one. He wouldn't stop until the main container was vacant.

It sounds straightforward, but "[w]within eighteen months, Dyrsmid was getting almost $5 million to the firm." (Clear, 2018, p. 196). He was effective because the positive routines he set up drove his determination and worked with his longing for progress

The most effective method to Build Your Resolve

Whether you accept determination as a restricted asset or something that can be 'refilled,' there are numerous ways it may very well be expanded.

Here are a few activities and ways of behaving that can assist with supporting your self-discipline

1. Strengthen your brain

"Mental uneasiness happens because you realise you are staying away from your obligations, so you take part in an interruption to lighten that distress."

The accompanying activities can assist with reinforcing your psyche, helping you to not take a simple choice, for instance, picking unfortunate dietary patterns or staying latent:

*Practice care reflection

To work on discretion and assist people with acting from expectation as opposed to propensity or hankering.

*Get sufficient rest

Physical and mental exhaustion can diminish resolve, so it's fundamental to keep up with energy levels by getting adequate and great quality rest every evening.

*Use food or wellness following applications

Following what we do or don't do can assist people with settling on better eating decisions and give consolation to get up and move by following development and exercise.

2. Develop your control

At the point when we trust our capacities and have confidence in our resolve, we are better ready to keep or recapture control

*Put forth clear and explicit objectives

An unmistakable comprehension of your objectives can assist with expanding inspiration and restraint.

*Separate enormous objectives into more modest, more reasonable assignments

More modest lumps of stir that develop into bigger objectives make it simpler to zero in on movement and remain persuaded.

*Work with an emotional wellness proficient

Advisors and advocates can give direction and backing in expanding self-discipline and building sound propensities.

3. Delivering your maximum capacity

At times our predispositions change how we see potential open doors and make us centre more around gambles than benefits. Pursuing choices in light of reason can assist us with understanding our maximum capacity alongside a kinder, more hopeful perspective on what we bring to the table.

*Challenge yourself

Propel yourself out of your usual range of familiarity by taking on complex yet not feasible errands. Practice and redundancy will help self-discipline.

*Practice self-sympathy

Be caring and understanding with yourself when you commit errors or stagger, and don't allow difficulties to deter you from proceeding to chip away at expanding your self-control.

*Get support from others

Encircle yourself with individuals who empower and uphold your endeavours to build your self-control.

It's a memorable fundamental that resolution resembles a muscle and that progress may not be quick or direct all of the time. Moreover, as actual activity, our psychological determination and poise can be fortified with training and pushing against apparent cutoff points.

Note that there is no "correct" measure of self-control, yet we should foster what is expected to carry on with a cheerful, solid life where we prosper.

Chapter 9

Basic ways of defining well-being and wellness objectives that will rouse you

Wellness objectives can be staggeringly rousing, yet without very arranged and practical goals, you might wind up baffled by an absence of anticipated results. Objective setting is a straightforward yet exceptionally strong game brain research tool. Goal setting assists you with further developing inspiration and responsibility, remaining fixed on what to achieve, and following your exhibition.

Defining Practical Wellness Objectives: Models to Consider

While defining wellness objectives, we frequently coincidentally sloppy our ways by being too excited or too aggressive in our objective setting, as per Dr. Galasso. Taking a quiet, sure way to deal with objective setting is best while defining individual objectives.

Truly ponder what you need to accomplish and the assets that you're ready to commit to your exercises, your eating regimen, and your recuperation [between practice sessions]. For example, the greatest snag that keeps the vast majority from making solid propensities isn't the craving to be better, but the "time" to do so, as indicated by Galasso. When laying out objectives, being open, genuine, and nonjudgmental about your assets is pivotal.

For instance, assuming you find your timetable is loaded with work, nurturing, and different responsibilities, then, at that point, rather than quickly focusing on working out at the exercise centre for an hour four times each week, think about your timetable, needs, and time requirements first.

Defining Shrewd Objectives

The Brilliant objective setting procedure is a famous technique for setting and getting a wide range of objectives, and it functions admirably for wellness. LifeTime ace fitness coach Danny Lord separates the parts of a Shrewd objective beneath.

*Explicit: Is your objective clear and defined?*Measurable: Might it at any point be followed? How might you be aware assuming you're gaining ground?

*Feasible: Is your objective testing yet doable?*Realistic: Is your objective pertinent to your life purpose?*Timely: Could you at any point relegate a date to consider yourself more responsible?

Done accurately, Shrewd objectives can be compelling, however, a great many people don't do it very right. He says Savvy objectives work best with process-arranged objectives as opposed to result objectives. Process objectives are centred around the genuine advances it takes to arrive at a particular result instead of zeroing in exclusively on the actual result.

For instance, an interaction-situated objective would be finishing a particular number of exercises each week. In the meantime, the objective is to lose a particular measure of weight. "The problem with utilising Shrewd objective defining for result situated objectives like weight reduction is that they are untidy and difficult to control. "It's not generally simple to know what's sensible or the specific period it will take to accomplish the objective."

Not gathering a major result in a situated objective can prompt debilitation — regardless of whether you're gaining huge headway — essentially because it didn't occur on your normal course of events. "I urge [my clients] to make an important, energising result-based objective and afterward a progression of Shrewd cycle objectives under that objective that will assist them with accomplishing the generally wanted objective.

Master Ways to Plan Practical Wellness Objectives at present
Utilise the direction underneath to create and achieve feasible wellness objectives that suit you and your way of life.

1. Use Perception to Track down Your 'Why'
Picturing your objectives kicks you off on your excursion, as per Louisa Nicola, overseer of Neuro Sports in Australia. Perception is a famous mental procedure that can assist with programming the brain and body to help fruitful objectives. Research recommends that envisioning yourself as fruitful can

prompt upgrades in execution, practice recurrence, concentration, and certainty.

Anything that you imagine, ought to be something you have an energetic outlook on and lines up with your qualities. "It's vital to imagine and have a greater longing while you're defining objectives. Ask yourself what gets you energised and gets a fire going in you. For what reason do you need this specific thing, and how significant is it to you?

This style of objective doesn't generally squeeze into the Shrewd system, yet it will assist with pushing you outside your usual range of familiarity to roll out an improvement, and it will be what to return to when inspiration runs short. "Your Savvy objective is meant to help this enormous enthusiastic 'why.'

2. Break Major Objectives Down Into More modest Parts

focusing on your objectives to keep away from a peculiarity called deferred limiting. "The more distance you make your objective, the less the award persuades conduct and the less dopamine [your brain] secretes in the quest for that objective," she says. She proposes making "set focuses" while heading to accomplishing your major objective that keeps your psyche and mind on target in quest for that objective.

For example, on the off chance that you have a significant weight reduction objective, put your focus on making gradual progress as opposed to zeroing in on the complete weight you need to lose. "Now and then, shedding 20 pounds is an incredibly long haul objective, yet it tends to be excessively lengthy for us to hold on to feel effective. Who recommends zeroing in on each pound of weight reduction, in turn, all things considered?

3. Create Everyday Objective Supporting Propensities

Bringing an end to down set focuses into propensities, or assignments you play out every day that help your objective's prosperity. For example, expanding your step count by 200 stages every day or guaranteeing you pack a high-protein and high-fibre nibble for work every day can uphold a general preparation objective.

Whenever you have clear assignments worked out every day to accomplish your month-to-month set focus, it reminds you to remain on track. Rehearsing centre activities can help, as well. Consider profound breathing, reflection, and leaving your telephone inactive for something like two hours per day to assist you with accomplishing your set focus.

4.Create Testing Yet Reachable Objectives

One explanation for why individuals don't accomplish their objectives is that they're either excessively simple or impossible — so finding a balance is fundamental. The research proposes that when individuals have scarcely unattainable objectives, they're more propelled and eager to pursue them, while objectives that are completely too far or too simple are excused before they even begin pursuing them.

Picking practices that meet your ongoing wellness level and guarantee you're not overlooking different parts of your well-being, like rest and nourishment. Keep an eating routine log to recognize areas of progress, and persistently track your exercises and movements. "It's essential to understand your body type, your wellness level, your way of life, and why you need to accomplish [your goal]. Base your objectives on your requirements — not external impacts. Thus, you can try not to overshoot or underrate your capacities.

5. Enjoy the Cycle

To put forth a practical objective, track down something that intrigues you and gives you pleasure, a confirmed fitness coach in New York. "There's not a glaringly obvious explanation to prepare for a long-distance race on the off chance that you disdain running." Finding something you appreciate improves the probability of you adhering to it since you're naturally persuaded to continue onward.

Research in the diary Brain Science and Wellbeing affirms that individuals will generally feel more sure and perform better assuming they appreciate what they're doing, and they're bound to continue to fabricate extra abilities that help their objectives.

I would urge individuals to contemplate the exercises they love and integrate them into their wellness objectives and schedule. For instance, somebody who loves golf could define an objective of doing a cardio exercise four times each week so they can at least walk 36 openings serenely in one day. If you're ready to integrate your wellness objectives into the exercises you normally appreciate doing day to day, week by week, or month to month, then, at that point, you have a lot higher likelihood of coming out on top.

6. Stay Positive

Remain peppy about hitting your objective — regardless of whether it takes more time than you'd like. Nothing works out coincidentally, no arrangement is awesome, and there will constantly be obstacles. "Recall that your period is inconsistent, and you will raise a ruckus around town sooner or later as long as you continue to work for it."

There might be minutes when you feel as though you miss the mark or on the other hand if the excursion is hard, don't make a move to be critical. Urge yourself to keep pushing ahead toward the fulfilment of your objective.

Fledgling Agreeable Wellness Objectives: Thoughts to Kick You Off

Now that you're outfitted with successful procedures for reasonable objective setting and prepared to get everything rolling, you might discover some motivation from the accompanying fledgling accommodating wellness objective thoughts:

1. For January, I will focus on three exercises each week — on Mondays, Wednesdays, and Fridays — for a sum of 13 exercises in the month.

2. I will require 8,000 stages each day for the principal seven-day stretch of January.

3. Every morning in January, I will hydrate.

4. By the end of Spring, I will finish something like 36 exercises.

5. I will pack a supplement-rich nibble for my day, something like three days a week for 30 days.

6. I will set a caution for clockwork during my business day to get up and take development breaks for 30 days.

7. I will learn and attempt another strength preparing development at regular intervals for the following half year.

8. I will build my means by 200 every day every week in February.

The most effective method to Get Your Wellness Ideas Rolling

To get your new wellness plan moving, get an organiser or schedule, and guide out day-to-day, week-by-week, month-to-month, and, surprisingly, yearly significant advances you need to take to help your goals. To assist you with remaining responsible, keep your objectives noticeable. "Record them on paper, express them without holding back, discuss them. Give them life."

Utilise a propensity tracker or a manual notes application to recognize whether you played out your errands as needed. Yet, sit back and relax on the off chance that you don't follow through with each job consistently — simply take up where you forget about and continue onward. Makes the biggest difference in consistency over the long run.

Assuming you can't finish your picked responsibilities reliably, it's ideal to reconsider them and why you may battle. "Was your Brilliant objective excessively forceful? Was it too severe to even think about squeezing into your way of life? Did you misjudge what you could focus on toward the beginning? Pose these inquiries as you work to define another more sensible objective.

At last, remember to place everything into a viewpoint, and be caring to yourself. There might be minutes when you believe you miss the mark or the excursion is hard, yet don't make a move to be critical. "Urge yourself to keep pushing ahead toward finishing your objective."

If you enjoyed this book kindly comment a Review Thank you.

amazon.com/author/bennettsbooks